I0439334

Apple Cider Vinegar Recipes for Health

by Rachel Jones

Disclaimer:

This book is for entertainment purposes. The publisher and author of this book are not responsible in any manner whatsoever for any damages arising directly or indirectly from use of the information in this book. Use this information at your own risk. The publisher and author disclaim any liabilities for damages caused by use of the information contained herein.

None of the claims in this book should be construed as medical advice. Consult with a medical professional prior to making any changes in your life that could impact your health.

Contents

The Many Faces of Apple Cider Vinegar

Anyone with even a passive interest in holistic health and home remedies has heard of apple cider vinegar. You can't take two steps in any direction in the natural health world without hearing about the many virtues of this versatile vinegar. Even if you don't buy into all the hype, there are a number of tangible benefits you can reap from adding apple cider vinegar to your diet. Apple cider vinegar can be used to improve your overall health, your complexion and may even be able to help you lose weight and better regulate your blood sugar.

Apple cider vinegar has been in use for thousands of years. It's been used as a condiment, a medicine and has even seen use on the battlefield as an antiseptic agent used to dress wounds. Our distant ancestors carried it on ships with them to fight scurvy and to preserve food. Japanese samurai drank it to give them strength as they headed into battle. Ancient kings used it to stay healthy and strong, while their queens used it as a health and beauty aid.

Cleopatra, the Queen of the Nile, is reputed to have consumed a glass of apple cider vinegar diluted with water after every meal in order to maintain her beauty and health. She also used it to win a bet she made with Marc Antony, a Roman politician and military general. Cleopatra bet Marc Antony that she could consume a fortune in a single meal. When Marc Antony took her up on the bet, the Queen took off one of her pearl earrings, made from the biggest pearls known to exist at the time, and dropped it into a cup of vinegar. The pearl dissolved, the Queen drank the vinegar, and the bet was won.

Move forward to modern times and apple cider vinegar is still a popular home remedy, used by people across the globe to improve their health. The health benefits of apple cider vinegar have been well-documented by those who use it over the years, but there have been relatively few scientific studies done to prove or disprove these benefits. The studies that have been done thus far are promising, but there aren't enough of them to draw many solid scientific conclusions.

One thing's for certain. People swear by apple cider vinegar as a remedy for almost any ailment imaginable. While the reality isn't quite what some people make of it, this pungent vinegar does have a number of therapeutic applications, both inside and outside of the body. The best part of all is it's completely natural and is safe for most people to consume in the amount required to reap the benefits.

What You Need to Know Before Buying Apple Cider Vinegar

The easiest way to obtain apple cider vinegar is to purchase it, either from a local grocer or health food store or from an online marketplace. Finding the right type of apple cider vinegar locally can be difficult, as many grocers don't stock the type of vinegar that has the most health benefits.

When buying apple cider vinegar, you're going to want to find vinegar that meets the following criteria:

- **It's organic.**
- **It's unpasteurized.**
- **It hasn't been filtered.**
- **It contains the mother.**

Organic apple cider vinegar is made from organic apples. This is preferable to vinegar made from conventionally-grown apple because conventional apples have been sprayed with pesticides, herbicides and all sorts of other chemical compounds by the time they reach the processing center. Trace amounts of these chemical compounds make it into the vinegar and are passed into your system when you consume the vinegar. The amount of chemicals in a teaspoon of vinegar is tiny and won't do much harm on its own, but over time these chemicals can build up in the body and may cause health problems later on down the road.

It's best to avoid the chemicals altogether instead of playing roulette with your future. Ensuring your vinegar is organic will ensure you aren't adding unwanted toxins to your body. After all, you're taking vinegar in an attempt to improve your health. Consuming anything but organic vinegar sort of defeats the purpose.

The next criteria you're going to want any apple cider vinegar you buy to meet is that it's unpasteurized and unfiltered. Raw apple cider vinegar contains a substance called the *mother of vinegar*. The mother contains healthy probiotic bacteria and is believed to be a big part of the reason why apple cider vinegar has so many health benefits. Pasteurization uses heat to kill all bacteria in the vinegar, and that includes the probiotic bacteria found in the mother. Vinegar that has been pasteurized has been rendered largely ineffective and isn't much more than water and acetic acid.

While perusing the shelves of your local grocery store, you may be tempted to buy filtered apple cider vinegar because it looks pretty. It's usually a beautiful translucent amber color and you can see through the container to the other side. If you were to head to the store to purchase apple cider vinegar without knowing what you were buying, you'd probably buy the filtered vinegar instead of the unfiltered stuff, which looks cloudy and murky. Filtered vinegar is clear because the mother has been filtered out of it. You end up with vinegar that looks good, but isn't anywhere near as good for you as the stuff that isn't filtered.

There are a number of brands that make unpasteurized, unfiltered, organic apple cider vinegar, but you aren't likely to find most of them on the shelves of your local grocery store. Health food stores usually carry them, but even there your options may be limited. If you don't have a health food store nearby, you can order apple cider vinegar online.

As far as brands go, Dynamic Health, Bragg and Fleishmann all make good vinegars that won't break the bank. Bragg has been in business since 1912 and is probably the gold standard when it comes to apple cider vinegar, but the other brands should work equally well.

Apple Cider Vinegar Pills

Apple cider vinegar pills are marketed to those who want to take advantage of the health benefits of apple cider vinegar without having to taste it while drinking or eating foods containing it. This would be great, if you could be sure of what the pills actually contain.

Researchers at the University of Arkansas took a look at some of the apple cider vinegar tablets sold in stores and the results were surprising. They looked at eight different brands and compared the tablet size, pH, acid content and label claims and found there was significant variability between the products. The labels were inconsistent and inaccurate and there were a number of unsubstantiated health claims made on the labels. The contents of the pills were so dubious, researchers questioned whether it was even apple cider vinegar in the pills (1).

The supplement market is largely unregulated in the United States, so it's all too easy to abuse the system. Manufacturers don't have to register supplements with the FDA or get approval prior to bringing supplements to market. Here's a direct quote from the FDA website:

"...FDA regulates dietary supplements under a different set of regulations than those covering "conventional" foods and drug products. Under the Dietary Supplement Health and Education Act of 1994 (DSHEA):

- The manufacturer of a dietary supplement or dietary ingredient is responsible for ensuring that the product is safe before it is marketed.

- FDA is responsible for taking action against any unsafe dietary supplement product after it reaches the market. "

That doesn't leave me with a warm, fuzzy feeling in my stomach about apple cider vinegar tablets, especially in light of what the researchers at the University of Arkansas found. I think I'll stick to adding apple cider vinegar to recipes.

Three Ways to Make Apple Cider Vinegar at Home

Apple cider vinegar is relatively inexpensive to purchase, so most people buy their apple cider vinegar instead of making it. A 32-ounce bottle will normally cost between $5 and $10. Be careful when buying vinegar online, because I've seen unscrupulous websites attempt to sell apple cider vinegar for much, much more. The kicker is it's the same vinegar that's available for less than $10 everywhere else. Also beware of suppliers selling artisanal vinegar in fancy bottles for premium prices. These vinegars may be better for cooking purposes, but aren't any better for you than the cheaper organic, unfiltered apple cider vinegars.

It'll probably cost you a bit more to make your own, but making it at home does afford you the advantage of having ultimate control over the ingredients that go into your vinegar. The best vinegar comes from organic apples that are ripe, but not overripe. Hand-selecting the apples yourself is the only way to ensure you're getting vinegar made from top-quality apples.

Apple cider vinegar is made via a process known as *fermentation*. This process is brought about as a result of the acetic acid bacteria in the mother acting upon the sugar found in apples. Acetic acid bacteria first ferment the sugar in apple cider into alcohol and then into acetic acid.

Acetic acid bacteria are required for fermentation because they're responsible for transforming alcohol into acetic acid. They can be added to the recipe by adding mother of vinegar (or vinegar containing the mother) or you can wait for the acetic acid bacteria that exist naturally on the vinegar to multiply. Adding mother of vinegar speeds the fermentation process up and helps ensure the right kind of bacteria grow inside the fermenting vessel.

Vinegar can be fermented in any container made of a non-reactive material. Glass, plastic and wood are the most common types of containers used to make apple cider vinegar. Most people make vinegar in glass containers because it's a benign material and is easy to clean. Plastic should be avoided because of the potential for it to leach chemicals into the vinegar, but that doesn't stop some people. Wood barrels are used by some manufacturers, but wood is rarely used by those looking to make vinegar at home.

Acetic acid bacteria require an aerobic environment in order to grow. Vinegar fermenting vessels are usually covered with a breathable material like cheesecloth that will keep insects out while allowing air to circulate into the container.

Sweet apples with high sugar content are the best apples to use to make vinegar. Green apples and other sour apple varieties don't work well because they don't contain enough sugar. Because the acid content in vinegar is directly related to the amount of sugar in the apples, the quality and acid content of homemade vinegar can vary greatly from batch to batch.

Homemade vinegar shouldn't be used for pickling purposes unless you've tested it and can be sure the acid content is at least 5%. Using vinegar with too low an acid content can result in foods that are tainted with botulism and other pathogens and are unsafe to eat. For this reason, it's best to use store-bought vinegar for pickling purposes because you can be sure of the acid content.

Apple Scrap Vinegar Recipe

The first method of making apple cider vinegar allows you to use apple scraps procured from apple you eat and making other recipes that call for apples. The peels and cores can be collected and frozen until you have enough.

You're going to need to gather the following supplies in order to make apple scrap vinegar:

- A wide-mouth jar.
- A piece of cheesecloth.
- A piece of twine or a large rubber band big enough to fit around the jar.
- A strainer.

The following ingredients are required:

- Apple scraps. These scraps can consist of the cores, skins and leftover flesh of any apples you use for other purposes.
- Filtered water.
- OPTIONAL: Mother of vinegar.

Here are the instructions for making apple scrap vinegar:

1. Lay the apple scraps out and let them air out until they turn brown. If you're using frozen scraps, this can take a while.
2. Rinse out a wide-mouth jar. The size of the jar you use depends on the quantity of apple scraps you have. Ideally, the jar will be almost completely full of scraps.
3. Fill the jar to within a couple inches of the top with apple scraps. Don't pack them in too tight.

4. Pour filtered water into the jar until it completely covers the apple scraps. Let it filter down into the scraps and continue adding water as necessary.

5. OPTIONAL: Add the mother of vinegar now, if you're going to add it.

6. Cover the jar with cheesecloth and secure it in place. The idea is to keep insects out while allowing fresh air to circulate through the jar.

7. Place the jar in a warm, dark place in your house and let it ferment. It'll take 4 to 6 weeks for the sugars in the apples to ferment into alcohol and then into the acids that make vinegar.

8. Taste-test the vinegar once every couple of days once it starts to smell acidic. When it tastes strong enough, strain the apple scraps away from the vinegar and discard the scraps.

9. Bottle the vinegar. It can be stored at room temperature.

The vinegar should be cloudy, as it will contain sediments from the apples and the mother. Don't attempt to get rid of all the sediment and the mother, as much of the health value of vinegar lies in the mother.

Whole Apple Cider Vinegar

Whole apples are used to make this vinegar. Vinegar made using this technique will be of higher quality than vinegar made using scraps because this vinegar uses the flesh of the apple instead of the scraps.

First, gather these supplies:

- A wide-mouth jar.
- A piece of cheesecloth.
- A piece of twine or a large rubber band big enough to fit around the jar.
- A strainer.

The following ingredients are required to make whole apple cider:

- Organic apples.
- Filtered water.
- OPTIONAL: Mother of vinegar.

Follow these directions to make whole apple cider vinegar:

1. Wash the apples.
2. Core and peel the apples. The peels and cores can be used to make apple scrap vinegar or they can be tossed in the compost heap.
3. Chop the apples into 1" to 2" chunks.
4. Let the apples sit until they start to turn brown.
5. Place the apples into a wide-mouth jar and add water to the jar until the apples are completely covered.

6. OPTIONAL: Add the mother of vinegar at this time, if you're going to add it.
7. Cover the mouth of the jar with cheesecloth and secure it in place.
8. Place the jar in a warm, dark area and leave it to ferment for 3 to 4 months. The liquid inside the jar will turn cloudy and the surface of the vinegar may become murky.
9. After 3 to 4 months have passed, strain the apples out of the vinegar. Place the vinegar back into the jar and recover it with cheesecloth. Let it ferment until the vinegar has soured to your liking. This can take another 1 to 2 months.
10. Once the vinegar has soured to your liking, bottle it in an airtight container.

You now have apple cider vinegar made from whole, organic apples. This vinegar can be used for most purposes vinegar is used for. Don't use it for food preservation without first testing the acidity, as the acid content can vary from batch to batch.

Vinegar from Cider Recipe

This is the most difficult of the apple cider vinegar recipes to make, but it can be used to make high-quality vinegar that tastes marginally better than the other two recipes. I'd say the quality of this vinegar is on par with the previous recipe using whole apples, with the main difference being you don't get as much sediment in this vinegar as you do when you use whole apples.

To make vinegar from cider, you're going to need the following items:

- A wide-mouth jar.
- Cheesecloth.
- A piece of twine or a large rubber band big enough to fit around the jar.

You're going to need the following ingredients:

- Organic apples.
- OPTIONAL: Mother of vinegar.

First, you're going to need to make apple cider. It takes approximately a third of a bushel of apples to make a gallon of apple cider. A third of a bushel weighs between 14 and 16 pounds.

Here are the instructions for making cider:

1. Wash the apples and crush them. You can pulse them in a blender or food processor if need be.
2. Place a piece of cheesecloth over a large bowl.
3. Pour the crushed apples onto the cheesecloth.
4. Make a bag out of the cheesecloth by folding up the corners.

5. Squeeze the apples inside the cheesecloth and let the apple juice drain into the bowl.
6. OPTIONAL: Add mother of vinegar to the apple cider at this time, if you plan on using it.

You now have the cider you need to make apple cider vinegar. The next step is to ferment the apple cider in an open container covered with cheesecloth until it becomes vinegar. This can take 1 to 3 months. Start checking the vinegar after a month and check it every couple of days thereafter until it's soured to your liking. Once the vinegar is ready, move it to an airtight container for storage.

This recipe can be made from store-bought apple cider if you don't want to make the cider yourself. For best results, use pure organic apple cider. Don't use apple juice because it has sugar and all sorts of other stuff added to it.

Why Not Take Apple Cider Vinegar By Itself?

The main reason most people prefer to take apple cider vinegar mixed into another food or beverage is the taste. It has a very strong flavor on its own and most people gag at the mere thought of taking apple cider vinegar on its own. The taste and smell of this pungent vinegar has been likened to "gym socks" and a "dirty locker room" by friends and family members who I've cajoled into trying it.

If you're one of the few people on this planet who actually likes the flavor of apple cider vinegar on its own, I commend you, but there's still good reason not to consume it undiluted. The acids in vinegar are strong enough to damage the teeth and consuming undiluted vinegar can compound the potential for damage. Undiluted vinegar can also damage the mucous membranes of the mouth, throat and esophagus.

The most common way people take apple cider vinegar is to dilute it with 8 ounces of water. That's the way most sources recommend taking it and that's the way I first started taking it. While diluting apple cider vinegar with water does make it semi-tolerable, it doesn't thin it out enough to allow you to forget you're drinking vinegar. It still burns a little going down and you still get the strong vinegar aftertaste, albeit not quite as strong as when it's undiluted.

Apple cider vinegar recipes add other ingredients to apple cider vinegar to make it more tolerable. I'm not going to lie to you and tell you that you won't be able to taste the vinegar at all. You'll still taste it a little, but it's much more palatable when it's combined with other ingredients that mask it.

The other benefit you get when adding apple cider vinegar to recipes is the ingredients of the recipe can be hand-picked to provide maximum therapeutic benefit. If you're going to drink something that's good for you, it might as well be packed full of good stuff, right?

Nutritional Information

Consuming a tablespoon or two of apple cider vinegar might be good for your health, but it's going to have minimal impact on your diet. Two tablespoons of apple cider vinegar amount to just over 6 calories and carry 0 glycemic load, so the total effect of apple cider vinegar on a normal diet in regards to caloric load and glycemic load is going to be next to nil.

The main mineral found in apple cider vinegar is potassium. A tablespoon of apple cider vinegar contains 11 mg of potassium. Apple cider vinegar also contains small amounts of calcium, manganese, iron, magnesium, phosphorus and sodium. It isn't believed to be a good source of vitamins, but some sources indicate it contains vitamins A, B1, B2, C and E.

The majority of apple cider vinegar is water, with H2O making up more than 90% of the total content of the vinegar. The acid content of apple cider vinegar usually hovers somewhere around 5%, with the majority of the acid being acetic acid. A handful of other acids are known to exist in apple cider vinegar as well, including malic acid, citric acid and lactic acid.

Apple cider vinegar also contains pectin, but it isn't clear how much of the pectin from the apples makes it into the finished vinegar.

Apple cider vinegar with the mother in it contains additional compounds pasteurized and filtered vinegar doesn't have. The mother is made primarily of cellulose and acetic acid bacteria, which are the bacteria responsible for turning the sugars in apple cider into the acids found in apple cider vinegar. The mother also contains enzymes that aid with digestion.

Apple Cider Vinegar Home Remedy Recipes

There are literally hundreds of ways apple cider vinegar is used as a natural remedy around the globe. You'd be hard-pressed to find a more versatile tool in the folk medicine lexicon. The uses outlined in this chapter are some of the more popular ways apple cider vinegar is used as a home remedy.

You may notice that none of the recipes call for adding apple cider vinegar to cooked dishes. The probiotic bacteria and enzymes in the mother will die when exposed to the high heats associated with cooking food. Apple cider vinegar can be used in culinary dishes that require cooking, but it will lose some of its effectiveness.

Be sure to only use organically grown ingredients in these recipes for best results. There's no telling what's been sprayed on conventionally-grown produce.

Alkalize the Body

The human body functions at a high level when it's slightly alkaline and health problems can start to occur if the body gets too acidic. When the body senses there is too much acid, it turns to the body's mineral reserves to help neutralize the acid. If the minerals aren't being replaced, these reserves can be depleted and all sorts of health problems can arise.

Since the Western diet is full of acidic foods, it's important to make sure you're consuming foods that are alkaline by nature to balance out the equation. The following foods are alkaline and can be added to your diet to aid with alkalinity:

- **Most raw vegetables (excluding corn, olives and winter squash).**
- **Most raw fruits (excluding blueberries, cranberries, currants and plums).**
- **Fresh herbs and spices.**
- **Sprouts.**
- **Some nuts, including almonds and chestnuts.**

It's important to note that a food's ability to form acids or alkalinity in the body has little to do with the acid content of the food itself. A food's alkalinity or acidity is determined by the residue the food leaves in the body once it has been digested.

While apple cider vinegar is acidic by nature, once it hits your stomach and is digested something strange happens. It becomes alkaline because of the ash content. Apple cider vinegar helps tilt your body towards alkalinity. This allows the body to more efficiently process the acids in the blood and may give your immune system a helping hand.

Alkalizing Lemon Water

Lemons contain citric acid, but contribute to alkalinity once consumed. Combining the alkalizing powers of lemons and apple cider vinegar creates a potent concoction for contributing to alkalinity in the body.

The following ingredients can be combined and consumed once or twice a day to help fight acidity:

- 8 ounces filtered water.
- 1 tablespoon apple cider vinegar.
- The juice of 2 lemons.
- ½ teaspoon cayenne pepper.

Cayenne peppers are one of the most alkalizing foods around. If you can't handle the pepper mixed into this drink, there are cayenne peppers pills that can be consumed instead.

Apple Alkaline Smoothie

Apples are alkalizing. So is apple cider. Combine the two with handful of other alkalizing ingredients and you get a tasty smoothie that helps balance your pH.

Gather the following ingredients:

- 3 apples, cored and quartered.
- 1 ripe nectarine, halved and pitted.
- 1 lime, peeled.
- 1 celery stick.
- 1 cup unsweetened apple juice or apple cider.
- 2 tablespoons apple cider vinegar.
- 5 to 10 ice cubes.

Add all of the ingredients to a blender and blend until smooth. Enjoy.

Sweetened Alkaline Lemonade

Instead of adding sugar, grapes are used to sweeten this lemonade to create an interesting fusion of flavors. Adding white sugar would tilt the balance toward acidity, but grapes are alkalizing, so you end up with an alkalizing (and refreshing) beverage.

Here are the ingredients you'll need:

- 2 cups water.
- 2 whole lemons, peeled.
- 2 cups seedless grapes.

Add all ingredients to a blender and blend on high until smooth. Serve chilled. If you don't like the pulp, you can pass the lemonade through a strainer, but removing the pulp will cause the loss of some of the health value.

Alkalizing Green Smoothie

Here's an alkalizing recipe that utilizes the power of a variety of leafy greens to alkalize the body. The apple cider vinegar adds even more alkalizing power, as do the coconut water and mint leaves.

Here are the ingredients you're going to need:

- 1 cup coconut water.
- Half a cucumber.
- 1 cup spinach.
- ¼ cup kale.
- ¼ cup collard greens.
- 5 mint leaves.
- 3 tablespoons lemon juice.
- 1 to 2 tablespoons apple cider vinegar.

Place all of the ingredients in a blender and blend until smooth. Drink immediately for best results.

Alkalizing Salad and Vinegar Dressing

Instead of giving you a recipe for salad, which I'm sure you already known how to make, this section contains a list of the numerous alkalizing vegetables that can be added to salad along with a handful of fruits you can also choose from. Pick your favorites and make an alkalizing salad that'll taste great and move the pH of your body in the right direction.

Here are the fruits and vegetables you can choose from:

- **Alfalfa.**
- **Beet greens.**
- **Beets.**
- **Broccoli.**
- **Cabbage.**
- **Carrots.**
- **Cauliflower.**
- **Celery.**
- **Chard greens.**
- **Chlorella.**
- **Collard greens.**
- **Cucumber.**
- **Dandelion greens.**
- **Eggplant.**
- **Fermented vegetables.**
- **Garlic.**
- **Green beans.**
- **Green peas.**
- **Kale.**
- **Kohlrabi.**

- **Lettuce.**
- **Mushrooms.**
- **Mustard greens.**
- **Nightshade vegetables.**
- **Nori.**
- **Onions.**
- **Peas.**
- **Peppers.**
- **Pumpkin.**
- **Radishes.**
- **Spinach.**
- **Spirulina.**
- **Sprouts.**
- **Sweet potatoes.**
- **Tomatoes.**
- **Watercress.**
- **Wheat grass.**

Combine the ingredients from this list in any way you'd like and then combine the following ingredients to make a tasty (and also alkalizing) dressing to top it with:

- 6 tablespoons extra virgin olive oil.
- 3 tablespoons apple cider vinegar.

Blend the oil and vinegar together and use it to top your salad. This dressing goes a little heavier on the vinegar than conventional vinaigrettes do. If it tastes too strong for your tastes, try cutting it back to 1 tablespoon of vinegar for every three tablespoons of oil, which is the standard for oil dressings.

If you want seasoned dressing, try adding ginger, garlic, sea salt or pretty much any herb you'd like. A half a teaspoon each of oregano, rosemary, basil and cumin will work wonders. Cayenne pepper is also alkalizing, so feel free to turn up the heat by adding it to the dressing as well.

Seasonal Allergy Relief

Spring time is a happy time of year.

Summer is almost upon us. The birds, bees and butterflies are fluttering about and plants are in full bloom. The spring season would be amazing, if it weren't for one little thing—allergies. OK, maybe for some of us that isn't such a little thing. For millions of people across the globe, allergy season is fraught with stuffy heads, coughing and itching and watering eyes, mouths, noses and throats.

Depending on where you live and what you're allergic to, allergy season can last for months. For some, the best months of the year are spent hiding out indoors and checking pollen reports before leaving the house.

Starting to take apple cider vinegar daily a few weeks prior to allergy season may get your body ready for the pollen you know is headed your way. Apple cider vinegar is believed to help boost your immune system and can help dampen the immune response when the pollen arrives. Apple cider vinegar probably isn't going to end your suffering altogether, but it might make things a tad more bearable during the normally difficult spring and summer months.

Allergy Relief Recipe

It's important to make sure the honey used for this recipe is from a local supplier because locally-sourced honey will have small amounts of pollen from plants that are blooming in your area in it. This is believed to help you build immunity against the pollen, as the honey won't have enough pollen in it to elicit a full-scale allergy attack, but may have enough to allow the body to adjust to it gradually if taken over time.

The following recipe can be used as a home remedy for allergies:

- 1 cup filtered water.
- 1 tablespoon apple cider vinegar.
- 2 tablespoons locally-sourced raw honey.

Gently warm the water and stir in the honey. Add the apple cider vinegar and drink the concoction while it's still warm.

Decongestant Steam Inhalation Recipe

If you're congested and are looking for almost instant relief, fill the sink up with steaming hot water and add the following ingredients:

- 5 drops eucalyptus essential oil.
- 5 drops tea tree oil.
- 3 tablespoons apple cider vinegar.

Drape a towel over your head and place your face above the steaming water. Be careful not to get so close that the steam burns you. Breathe deeply and inhale the steam for 5 to 10 minutes. Do this when you first wake up and again right before bed.

Stinging Nettle Tea

Stinging nettle is an interesting plant. Walk through a patch of stinging nettle and let it come in contact with exposed skin and you're in for a world of hurt, as the itching and burning can get pretty intense. Make a tea of it and you might end up singing its praises for its ability to relieve allergies.

There are studies that show stinging nettle to be effective at relieving allergies. One study that used stinging nettle extract found it stopped inflammatory events that led to allergic reactions in the body (2). Another study found freeze-dried stinging nettle to be effective in relieving at least some of the symptoms of allergic rhinitis (3).

Stinging nettle tea can be combined with apple cider vinegar to create a tea that might be able to eliminate many of the symptoms associated with allergies. Gather the following ingredients in order to make stinging nettle tea:

- 2 tea bags containing stinging nettles.
- 2 cups water.
- 1 tablespoon apple cider vinegar.
- 2 tablespoons raw honey (locally sourced).

Follow these directions to make stinging nettle tea:

1. Bring the water to a boil.
2. Place the tea bags in the pot.
3. Turn off the heat and let the tea steep for 15 to 20 minutes.
4. Stir in the honey and the apple cider vinegar.

You've now got tea that combines three of the most well-known natural allergy relief solutions. It's probably best to consume this tea first thing in the morning and then again later on in the day if symptoms start to arise.

Rooibos Ginger Tea

Rooibos tea, also known as *red bush tea*, is a caffeine-free tea that contains *quercetin*. The quercetin in the tea is thought to block the release of histamine in the body, which is a chemical the body releases when it senses an allergen. Quercetin is also found in apples, so it's in apple cider vinegar as well.

Ginger is also an antihistamine, so it was added to this recipe to further mute the body's immune response.

In order to make rooibos tea, gather the following ingredients:

- 2 teaspoons rooibos tea.
- 1 cup water.
- 1 teaspoon grated ginger.
- 1 tablespoon apple cider vinegar.

Here are the directions:

1. Bring the water to a boil.
2. Remove the water from the heat and add the ginger and rooibos tea to it.
3. Let it steep for 10 minutes.
4. Strain the tea to remove the rooibos tea and ginger.
5. Add the apple cider vinegar.
6. Drink while warm or pour it over ice.

If you want to sweeten this tea, use locally sourced organic honey.

Bad Breath

There are as many home remedies for bad breath as there are causes of it. Most of the remedies simply seek to mask the foul odors emanating from the mouth and do little to actually get rid of the bacteria that the likely culprit. As soon as the remedy is no longer in your mouth, your breath will be right back to being ripe.

A simple solution of a tablespoon of apple cider vinegar mixed into a cup of water can be gargled to get rid of the bacteria that reside on the back of the tongue. These bacteria are often the culprit when it comes to bad breath. Don't swallow the solution you gargled with, as it could be teeming with bad bacteria. Don't swish this solution around your mouth. The acids in the vinegar can damage tooth enamel. Rinse your mouth out thoroughly after using apple cider vinegar to gargle with and avoid brushing your teeth for at least 30 minutes.

Some sources recommend using apple cider vinegar mixed with water and other ingredients as an antibacterial mouthwash. This is not a good idea because of the propensity for enamel damage.

Another remedy you can try is dipping a damp toothbrush into baking soda and using it to brush your teeth. There could be food and bacteria trapped in gum pockets that are causing the bad smell and the baking soda will go a long way toward neutralizing them. Make sure you brush as far back on your tongue as you can get.

One more trick you can use is to chew on aromatic spices throughout the day. Cloves and fennel seed can both be chewed to help get rid of bad breath. Steer clear of gum and mints that contain sugar because they'll feed the bacteria and ultimately make your breath worse. The spices have antibacterial properties, so they'll help eliminate bacteria from the mouth instead of helping them grow.

When all else fails, combine a tablespoon of apple cider vinegar with 8 ounces of water and drink it once a day. Bad breath can arise due to internal imbalances and apple cider vinegar may be able to help rebalance your body toward good health and eliminate the bad breath from the inside out.

Green Tea Breath Booster

Green tea is a powerful source of polyphenol antioxidants. It's known to benefit the heart and to help boost the immune system. According to scientists at the Israel School of Technology, a polyphenol known as EGCG is able to eliminate halitosis by modifying odorant sulfur components (4). Green tea doesn't just help with bad breath at the moment—it takes the fight to the bacteria that cause bad breath and helps eliminate them while improving overall dental health.

Add a tablespoon or two of apple cider vinegar to a cup of green tea to combine the antibacterial powers of the tea with the vinegar. Steep a cinnamon stick in the tea and add a few sprigs of mint for an even more potent punch.

Here are the ingredients for the Green Tea Breath Booster:

- 1 cup water.
- 1 green tea bag.
- 1 to 2 tablespoons apple cider vinegar.
- 1 cinnamon stick.
- 2 mint sprigs.

Follow these directions:

1. Bring the water to a boil.
2. Remove it from the heat and place the green tea bag into the water.
3. Add the cinnamon stick.
4. Let the tea steep for 10 minutes.

5. Remove the cinnamon stick and the green tea bag.
6. Add the apple cider vinegar and mint sprigs.
7. Drink while warm.

P a g e | 47

Aloe Apple Juice

Aloe vera packs a potent one-two punch when it comes to bad breath. Pure aloe gel is antifungal and antiviral, so it's able to combat the microorganisms that cause bad breath in the mouth. Aloe juice is able to ease acid indigestion once ingested, which is one of the causes of bad breath.

The apple juice isn't just in this recipe for flavor. The quercetin in apples inhibits the growth of bacteria in the mouth and helps strengthen the gums.

Here are the ingredients:

- 1 cup fresh unsweetened apple juice.
- 1 cup aloe vera juice.
- 1 tablespoon apple cider vinegar.

The directions for this recipe are simple. Mix the ingredients together and drink the juice.

Blood Pressure

Lifestyle choices often play a large role when it comes to blood pressure. Smoking, drinking, eating unhealthy foods and sitting on the couch (or behind a desk) all day can all lead to hypertension. Doctors tend to want to prescribe medications to lower blood pressure, but a handful of lifestyle changes may enable you to lower your blood pressure naturally and without risk of the side effects associated with BP medications.

Here are some of the changes you can make in your life that might lower your blood pressure:

Lose weight. If you're overweight, shedding those excess pounds can go a long way toward reducing blood pressure.

Eat healthy foods. Eat more fruit, whole grains, vegetables and fermented dairy products. Skip the salt, sugar, red meats and processed foods. Foods containing potassium can help lower blood pressure in some individuals, so eat more bananas and apples.

Hit the gym (or get some other form of daily exercise). 30 minutes to an hour of exercise a day has been shown to lower blood pressure. It can also help those on the cusp of becoming hypertensive avoid reaching dangerously high levels. According to some sources, aerobic exercise can reduce systolic blood pressure by as much as 5 points and may eventually allow you to reduce the amount of hypertension medications you're taking (5).

Stop drinking. Well, at least slow down a bit. If you're drinking more than 1 to 2 drinks a day, you can probably lower your blood pressure a bit by cutting back to the recommended minimum. And no, a 40-ounce beer doesn't count as one drink. One drink is defined as 1 ½ ounces of hard liquor, 12 ounces of beer or 5 ounces of wine.

Stop smoking. Smoking almost instantly raises your blood pressure and keeps it elevated for a significant amount of time. If you're smoking half a pack a day, you're probably keeping your blood pressure elevated above where it should be for most of the day.

Cut back on the coffee. Some people are more sensitive to caffeine than others and can see as much as a 10 point spike in their blood pressure after drinking something with caffeine in it. If you're one of those people, cutting out the coffee can lower your blood pressure significantly.

Stop stressing out. I know, easier said than done, right? Try to keep stress to a minimum and you might lower your blood pressure as a result.

•••

The querticin in apples has been shown to lower blood pressure. Apple cider vinegar also contains potassium, which helps the body handle salt.

It's unlikely apple cider vinegar alone will have much effect on blood pressure, but it may have a synergistic effect when combined with the lifestyle changes laid out above. The recipes in this section are most likely to help those who aren't yet hypertensive and are living a healthy lifestyle.

Never assume lifestyle or dietary changes will lower your blood pressure or will allow you to stop taking blood pressure medication. Be aware it may be dangerous to make certain dietary or lifestyle changes while on blood pressure medication. The drop in blood pressure associated with certain dietary or lifestyle changes could combine with the drop in blood pressure associated with the medication and cause your BP to dip too low.

Discuss any changes you plan on making with your doctor in advance of actually making the change. Your doctor can assist you in making healthy choices that are right for your current physical state.

Banana & Greens Smoothie

According to the American Heart Association, natural sources of potassium play an important role in controlling blood pressure because they help the body regulate the effects of sodium. Bananas and spinach are both high in potassium, with a medium banana containing 422 mg of potassium and a cup of spinach containing 167 mg of potassium.

This smoothie combines bananas and spinach with a tablespoon of vinegar to provide maximum effect.

Here are the ingredients you'll need:

- 1 cup spinach.
- 2 bananas.
- 1 cup almond milk.
- 5 ice cubes.
- 1 tablespoon apple cider vinegar.

Add everything to a blender and blend until smooth. Consume immediately.

Pepper Tomato Juice

The heat from the cayenne pepper may have a positive effect on blood pressure and the lycopene in the tomato juice is an antioxidant that could further lower blood pressure. If the cayenne pepper doesn't go down smoothly enough for your tastes, try adding cinnamon instead. Cinnamon is another compound that's been shown to reduce blood pressure.

The following recipe may help lower blood pressure:

- 8 ounces of low-sodium tomato juice or V8.
- 1 tablespoon of apple cider vinegar.
- 1 teaspoon cayenne pepper.

Add all of the ingredients to a cup and stir until blended. Drink immediately for best results.

Pomegranate-Mango Smoothie

Pomegranate juice has been shown to reduce blood pressure when consumed long-term. One study found supplementing the diet with pomegranate juice helped reduce systolic blood pressure in participants by 12% (6). Mangoes are also supposed to have a positive effect on blood pressure, which is why they've been added to this smoothie.

Here are the ingredients you're going to need:

- 1 cup pomegranate juice.
- 2 mangoes.
- 1 tablespoon apple cider vinegar.
- Raw honey, to taste.
- A handful of ice cubes.

Add all of the ingredients to a blender and blend until smooth. Drink immediately.

Purple Potato Salad

Potatoes have a bad reputation in the world of healthy living. For the most part, it's well-deserved. They're heavy on carbs and contain a lot of starch. This has led most healthy living experts to vilify potatoes, placing them on the very short list of vegetables that aren't good for you to consume regularly.

A recent study may end up breaking the stereotype potatoes have garnered as an unhealthy food. A research report presented at the 242nd National Meeting & Exposition of the American Chemical Society revealed that a couple servings a day of potatoes cooked in a healthy manner reduces both systolic and diastolic blood pressure without leading to weight gain. The potatoes used in the study were purple-skinned potatoes, but scientists think other potatoes would have a similar effect (7).

The key to using potatoes to your benefit instead of to your detriment is to cook them in a healthy manner. Steer clear of the butters and fats normally used to cook potatoes and boil or microwave them instead of frying them, which eliminates a large amount of the health value.

The following recipe calls for purple-skinned potatoes, but if you're concerned with the health value of the potatoes, you can substitute sweet potatoes into the recipe. Most health experts agree sweet potatoes are good for you.

Gather the following ingredients to make this potato salad:

- 1 pound baby purple-skinned potatoes.

- 2 cloves garlic, minced.
- ½ of a medium onion.
- ½ cup chopped celery.
- ¼ cup chopped dill pickles.
- 1 cup plain yogurt.
- ½ tablespoon yellow mustard.
- 5 tablespoons apple cider vinegar.
- ½ teaspoon red pepper flakes.
- ½ teaspoon sea salt.
- ½ teaspoon cayenne pepper.

Follow these directions to make purple potato salad:

1. Place the potatoes in a microwave-safe dish and cover the dish.
2. Microwave on high for 10 to 15 minutes, or until potatoes are soft.
3. Let the potatoes cool and cut them into bite-sized cubes.
4. Place the cubed potatoes into a bowl with the rest of the ingredients and toss until the ingredients are mixed and the potatoes are coated.
5. Chill and serve.

Blood Sugar

There have been a number of studies done that seem to indicate apple cider vinegar is able to help regulate the rise in blood sugar associated with eating a meal that's high in complex carbs. These studies have linked consumption of vinegar to both lowered blood glucose levels and lowered insulin response after a meal.

The most notable studies are those conducted by Carol S. Johnson and her team at Arizona State University. They've conducted 5 studies, and all of the studies have shown positive results.

Here's a quick rundown of what the studies have revealed:

- The first study showed consuming apple cider vinegar after a meal consisting of a bagel and orange juice lowered insulin response and blood glucose in both diabetic and prediabetic study participants (8).
- The next study found that both vinegar and peanut products were capable of reducing glucose response after a high-glycemic load meal (9).
- The third study showed that consuming vinegar and cheese in the evening before bed resulted in reduced blood sugar when the participants woke up in the morning (10).
- Another study found consuming vinegar before a meal reduced postprandial glycemia by up to 20% (11).

- In yet another study, daily consumption of vinegar was shown to work to lower fasting glucose concentrations over a period of 12 weeks (12).

There have been a handful of other studies that have shown similar results. While using apple cider vinegar as a means of reducing blood sugar looks promising, there is the potential of vinegar interacting with prescription medications. Consult with your doctor as to what the acceptable dosage of apple cider vinegar for attempting to lower your blood sugar would be.

Kale and Lima Bean Salad

According to the Joslin Diabetes Center, soluble fiber helps lower cholesterol and improves blood glucose control if eaten in large amounts. It also aids with helping you feel full, so you don't overeat (13).

Both kale and lima beans are high in soluble fiber. A cup of kale contains nearly 2 grams of soluble fiber and half a cup of lima beans contains more than 2 grams. A single lima bean and kale salad can provide you with more than 4 grams of soluble fiber.

Here are the ingredients you're going to need to make this salad:

- 1 cup kale, stemmed and chopped.
- ½ cup lima beans.
- 1 tablespoon fresh lemon juice.
- 4 tablespoons extra virgin olive oil.
- 1 tablespoon apple cider vinegar.
- 1 garlic clove, minced.

Here are the directions for making this salad:

1. Place the lima beans in a bowl. Cover them with water and leave them to soak overnight.
2. Drain the water away from the beans.
3. Place the beans in a saucepan and cover them with water.
4. Bring the water to a boil. Back the heat off until the water is simmering and let the beans cook for an hour, or until they're soft.
5. Drain the water away from the beans.

6. Place the kale in a bowl. Add the lemon juice, olive oil and apple cider vinegar to the bowl and massage it into the kale.
7. Stir in the garlic.
8. Stir the lima beans into the salad.
9. Place the salad into the fridge and let it chill for at least 15 minutes.

Steamed Broccoli & Vinegar

We've already discussed soluble fiber and how it relates to blood sugar. Broccoli is high in soluble fiber, but that isn't its only benefit. It also contains enzymes known as *sulforaphanes* that may protect or even reverse the damage done by high blood sugar (14).

Don't use frozen broccoli to make this recipe, as research has shown broccoli that's blanched at high heat and then frozen lacks the enzymes required to form sulforaphane (15). Cooking broccoli at high heat destroys much of the sulforaphane content. Steaming is one of the few methods that doesn't eliminate much of the sulforaphane from broccoli (16), so that's the method used in this recipe.

Here are the ingredients needed for steamed broccoli and vinegar:

- ½ pound broccoli florets.
- 1 tablespoon apple cider vinegar.
- 2 tablespoons extra-virgin olive oil.
- A pinch of salt.
- A pinch of pepper.

Here are the directions:

1. Wash the broccoli and break it up into florets.
2. Steam the broccoli in a steamer for 6 to 8 minutes.
3. Let the broccoli cool for 5 minutes and move it to a large bowl.

4. Add the olive oil, salt and pepper to the bowl and toss the broccoli in it until it's thoroughly coated.
5. Drizzle the vinegar over the broccoli right before serving it.

Cancer

NOTE: Apple cider vinegar is not a proven treatment for diagnosed cases of cancer. It has been shown to have antitumor properties in a select few studies done on animals in a laboratory setting, but should not be used to attempt to treat an existing case of cancer.

Studies have shown vinegar may be able to kill cancer cells by inducing *apoptosis* (17). When apoptosis occurs, the cells basically self-destruct and are quickly cleared out of the body. The studies that have been done thus far on lab animals have used types of vinegar other than apple cider vinegar, so it isn't known for sure whether apple cider vinegar has the same antitumor effect.

While the initial studies are promising, a lot more research needs to be done.

To be clear, the recipes in this section are not in any way, shape or form a cure for cancer. They aren't a treatment for existing cancer either. They may be able to help the body prevent cancer cells from forming and may slow the growth of cancer, but much more research is warranted before any solid conclusions can be drawn. The stakes are high with cancer, so never attempt to treat or cure cancer with home remedies.

If you or a loved one has cancer or you suspect you or a loved one has cancer, it's time to get in to see a doctor immediately. Time is of essence and the longer you wait, the less likely you are to survive. I can't stress enough how important it is to get in and get an early diagnosis. At the very least, it'll allow you to stop stressing out about something you thought could be cancer. If there is cancer in your body, early diagnosis could be the difference between a quick outpatient procedure and years spent battling this invasive and deadly disease.

Discuss the risks and benefits of adding new recipes to your diet prior to adding them. This is especially important if you're currently undergoing treatment, as dietary changes could interfere with chemotherapy and other cancer treatments.

Lemon Cinnamon Green Tea

Green tea contains a number of *polyphenols* and *flavonoids* that have been shown to have strong antioxidant capabilities. *Catechins* in particular are garnering notice in the scientific community for their ability to ward off cancer. Green tea has been shown in laboratory settings to prevent the development of certain types of cancer and studies on people that track food consumption have shown regular consumption of green tea lowers the risk of certain types of cancer (18).

When it comes to lemons and lemon juice, there's a lot of misinformation floating around. There's an e-mail floating around that claims lemons, lemon juice and ground up lemon rind are capable of eradicating cancer in the body. While that simply isn't true, lemons do contain flavonoids and other antioxidant compounds that scavenge free radicals in the body. This ability to scavenge free radicals may help prevent cancer by preventing the cell damage that leads to the formation of cancerous cells, but it's far from a cure for cancer.

Cinnamon may also have some anticancer properties. City of Hope researchers tested cinnamon extract and found it interferes with a special protein cancer uses to establish a blood supply to growing tumors (19).

Gather the following ingredients to make this tea:

- 1 cup water.
- 2 tablespoons crushed green tea leaves.
- ½ teaspoon ground cinnamon.
- 3 tablespoons fresh lemon juice.

- 1 tablespoon apple cider vinegar.
- Raw honey, to taste.

Here are the directions for making the tea:

1. Heat the water to a boil.
2. Turn off the heat and add the crushed green tea leaves to the water.
3. Add the cinnamon and fresh lemon juice. Stir in the honey.
4. Let the tea steep for 10 minutes.
5. Strain out the tea leaves and place the tea in a cup.
6. Add the apple cider vinegar.
7. Drink while lukewarm. Do not reheat the tea because it can kill the probiotic bacteria in the vinegar.

Apple Cinnamon Cider w/ Apple Cider Vinegar

There really is something to the old adage, "An apple a day keeps the doctor away." Apples are packed to the brim with vitamins, nutrients and phytochemicals that improve health and help the body fight off disease.

According to the American Institute for Cancer Research, apples contain antioxidants and other chemical compounds that prevent oxidative damage to cells, prevent cancer from starting, stop the growth of existing tumors and promote the death of cancer cells (20). Consumption of apples may lead to less risk of developing a number of cancers, including prostate, breast, lung, liver and colon cancer (21).

Fresh apple cider contains many of the same phytochemicals you get when you eat a raw apple. It's still a good idea to eat an apple a day even if you consume this recipe because apples provide a more balanced nutritional profile.

This is a good recipe for those looking to mask the taste of apple cider vinegar because apple cider does a fairly good job of covering up the taste of apple cider vinegar. There's still a bit of aftertaste of vinegar, but it isn't anywhere near as bad as when you take vinegar diluted in water.

Here are the ingredients you'll need:

- 2 cups apple cider.
- 1 teaspoon ground cinnamon.
- 1 tablespoon raw honey.

- 1 tablespoon apple cider vinegar.

Follow these directions to make apple cinnamon cider:

1. Gently warm the apple cider. Don't heat it up too much.
2. Stir in the raw honey.
3. Add the cinnamon and stir it in.
4. Let the cider cool and add the vinegar.
5. The cider can be served lukewarm or you can chill it and serve it cold.

Blueberry Chia Seed Pudding

Blueberries are an excellent source of fiber, vitamin C and vitamin K. Chemical compounds known as *anthocyanins* give blueberries their dark blue color and may play a role in slowing tumor growth and counterbalancing oxidative damage in the body. In a laboratory setting, blueberry juice has been shown to block the migration of a certain type of breast cancer cells and blueberry extract was shown to reduce the size of tumors (19).

Chia seeds contain *omega-3 fatty acids*, which are sorely lacking in the Western diet. Omega-3's are good for your overall health and are tasked with reducing inflammation in the body. Inflammation does damage to healthy cells and is believed to be one of the reasons cancer cells start to grow (22). Oil extracted from chia seeds has been show to induce apoptosis in cancer cells in a laboratory setting (23). Chia seeds are also high in fiber, packing in 10 grams of fiber per ounce. The results of studies on fiber have been mixed in regards to fiber's ability to fight most cancers, but fiber is an essential part of a healthy diet (24).

To make blueberry chia seed pudding, you're going to need the following ingredients:

- ¼ cup chia seeds.
- 1 cup almond milk.
- ½ cup organic blueberries.
- ½ teaspoon vanilla extract.
- ½ teaspoon ground cinnamon.
- ½ teaspoon ground cardamom.

- Raw honey, to taste.
- 1 teaspoon apple cider vinegar.

Here are the directions for making this pudding:

1. Add all of the ingredients except the chia seeds to a blender and blend until smooth.
2. Place the chia seeds in a bowl and stir the blueberry pudding mixture in with the seeds.
3. Refrigerate for 15 minutes and whisk vigorously.
4. Place the pudding back in the fridge and leave it there overnight.
5. Whisk again in the morning. More almond milk can be added if the pudding is too thick for your tastes.

Clear Out Candida

Candida overgrowth is a fungal infection that usually starts in the gut and can spread to the rest of the body. Small amounts of candida yeasts exist naturally in the gut, lungs, bladder mouth, genitals and other areas where there are mucus membranes. They aren't supposed to grow out of control until you pass away, at which time they're tasked with breaking the body down and helping it decompose.

Under normal conditions, candida lives in harmony with the other microorganisms in the body and is kept in check by probiotic bacteria. It doesn't become problematic until something happens to upset this balance and candida is able to grow unchecked. Candida infections usually start in the gut, but can perforate the intestines and make their way into the bloodstream. Once in the bloodstream, candida can travel throughout the body and have the ability to wreak havoc anywhere it goes.

The following symptoms are often associated with candida infection:

- **Aches and pains.**
- **Acid reflux.**
- **Acne and other skin problems.**
- **Bloating.**
- **Constipation.**
- **Coughing.**
- **Cravings for sugar and simple carbohydrates.**
- **Diarrhea.**
- **Fatigue and weariness.**
- **Gas.**

- **Genital itching.**
- **Genital yeast infections.**
- **Headaches and migraines.**
- **Low sex drive.**
- **Mood swings.**
- **Rectal itching.**
- **Sore throat.**
- **Thrush.**
- **Vaginitis.**

These are just some of the many symptoms of candida overgrowth. Once the infection reaches your bloodstream, symptoms can pop up anywhere. Candida can negatively impact the digestive, nervous, cardiovascular, lymphatic and skeletal system, and can overburden the immune system, opening the body up to attack from harmful bacteria and pathogens.

The most well-known candida infection is the vaginal yeast infection. This type of infection can be passed between partners via sexual contact and isn't limited to just women. Men can suffer candida infection as well. The symptoms in men might be minor or even non-existent, and a male partner can continuously pass a yeast infection back to the female in the relationship if his infection is left untreated.

A healthy immune system and gut is vital to keeping candida in check. One of the major causes of candida overgrowth is the use of antibiotics to treat other problems. Antibiotics kill the good bacteria in the body along with the bad. Candida yeasts are able to resist most antibiotics, so they're likely to be the first to grow to replace healthy bacteria lost to antibiotics.

Taking probiotic supplements and eating probiotic foods like kefir and fermented vegetables can help replace the healthy bacteria before candida can step in to replace them. Avoid foods containing sugars and simple carbohydrates because these foods feed candida. Processed foods and foods containing trans fats are also bad because they weaken the immune system and anything with gluten should be avoided because it can do further damage to both the intestines and the immune system.

Replace bad cooking oils containing trans fats with unrefined organic coconut oil. Coconut oil can help the body battle candida because it's antifungal by nature. It also gives the immune system a healthy hand and aids with digestion. Some people take a tablespoon or two of coconut oil per day as a supplement.

Garlic Tea

Apple cider vinegar and garlic both have antifungal properties. Lemon juice helps your liver function at a high level and is also mildly antifungal. All three ingredients can be combined to make a tea that doesn't taste great, but can be used to help the body fight candida infection.

Here are the ingredients you're going to need:

- 1 quart filtered water.
- 4 garlic cloves, minced.
- The juice from 2 lemons.
- 5 tablespoons apple cider vinegar.

Follow these directions to make the tea:

1. Bring the water to a boil.
2. Remove the pot from the heat and add the lemon juice and garlic cloves to the pot.
3. Let it steep for 30 minutes.
4. Pour the water through a strainer to remove the garlic.
5. Add the apple cider vinegar to the tea and stir it in.

This tea can be consumed warm or cold. Don't heat it up too much with the apple cider vinegar in it or you'll kill the probiotic bacteria. Drink 2 to 3 cups of tea per day while trying to rid yourself of candida.

Fermented Dilly Carrots

Fermented vegetables contain probiotic bacteria, so consuming them may help the body crowd out candida bacteria in the gut. Candida yeasts feed on sugars and lacto-fermented foods like fermented dilly carrots are low on sugar because the lactobacteria have already partially digested the sugars as they develop. They provide the body with nutrition and energy without further promoting the growth of candida.

Here are the ingredients you're going to need to make fermented dilly carrots:

- 6 medium carrots.
- 2 garlic cloves.
- 2 sprigs of fresh dill.
- A starter culture packet.
- 1 tablespoon unrefined sea salt.
- 3 cups filtered water.

You're also going to need a fermenting container. Traditionally, vegetables have been fermented in canning jars, but there are specialty fermenting jars available that make fermenting a breeze. Foods have to be fermented in an anaerobic environment and these specialty jars do a great job of keeping oxygen out while allowing the gases created during fermentation to escape the jar.

Here are the instructions for making dilly carrots:

1. Wash the carrots.
2. Peel them and cut them into sticks.
3. Chop the dill.

4. Peel and mince the garlic cloves.

5. Add the carrots, dill and garlic cloves to the fermenting jar.

6. Mix the sea salt and the water to make brine. Pour the brine over the top of the carrots. Get rid of any air bubbles in the carrots. Air bubbles create pockets in the jar in which the carrots can spoil.

7. Place a weight in the jar to keep the carrots below the surface of the brine. The weight can be anything that's made of a non-reactive material like glass or smooth stone and is large enough to prevent the carrots from floating to the surface. This is critical because any carrots allowed to float to the surface of the brine will be exposed to oxygen and could spoil.

8. Add more brine, as necessary, to ensure the weight is covered with brine. Leave an inch of airspace at the top of the container.

9. Cover the container and seal it so it's airtight. If you're using a specialty fermenting container, follow the manufacturer's instructions for sealing the container.

10. Store the container in a dark place at room temperature for 5 to 7 days.

11. After 5 days, check the carrots daily to see if they're done. Once they start to taste and smell sour, they're ready to eat and can be moved to the fridge. If they start to smell rotten or mold forms at the top of the container, do not eat the carrots.

A tablespoon or two of apple cider vinegar can be added to the carrots at the time you eat them. Do not add the vinegar before fermenting the carrots because it can inhibit the growth of probiotic bacteria in the container.

Lower Cholesterol

Low-density lipoprotein (LDL) is considered bad cholesterol because it can stick to your arteries. LDL cholesterol sticks to the walls of arteries and white blood cells attach themselves to the LDL cholesterol, which eventually results in arteries clogged with a substance known as *plaque*. Too much plaque can result in strokes, heart disease and a variety of other health problems.

To reduce cholesterol naturally, go easy on the red meat, chicken and dairy. Foods that come from animals have cholesterol in every cell, so trimming off the fat won't cut it. It's also as good idea to avoid foods that are high in trans fats, so processed foods and junk food is out of the question. Foods rich in soluble fiber help the body eliminate cholesterol, so go heavy on the beans, okra and oats. A handful of almonds per day can also help since they have sterols that will further reduce cholesterol.

A couple studies have shown vinegar to be effective in lowering cholesterol in both rats and in humans. The initial results are promising, but more research is warranted. Don't expect any miracles from apple cider vinegar, but it may be able to help a little.

Green Tea w/ Flaxseed

Green tea contains compounds known to lower LDL cholesterol. Flaxseed has also been shown to lower LDL cholesterol in healthy young adults (25).

The following recipe combines ground flax seed, green tea and apple cider vinegar:

- 1 cup water.
- 1 green tea bag.
- 1 teaspoon ground flaxseeds.
- 1 tablespoon apple cider vinegar.

Here are the directions for making green tea with flaxseeds:

1. Bring the water to a boil. Remove the pot from the heat.
2. Add the flaxseeds to the water.
3. Steep the tea for 30 minutes.
4. Let the tea cool to lukewarm before adding the apple cider vinegar. Stir it in and drink the tea.

Walnut & Pear Salad

Walnuts contain polyunsaturated fatty acids, which are good fats the body needs. A handful of walnuts a day is believed to reduce the risk of heart disease, as long as the nuts haven't been salted (26).

Pectin is a water-soluble fiber that has the ability to bind to cholesterol while it's still in the stomach, effectively preventing it from making its way into the bloodstream (27). Apples are known for their pectin content, but pears contain even more pectin than apples, which makes them an effective home remedy for helping lower cholesterol.

Gather the following ingredients to make walnut and pear salad:

- 1 medium pear, cored and sliced.
- 2 cups salad greens.
- ¼ cup diced onions.
- 3 tablespoons unsalted, halved walnuts.
- 2 tablespoons pear nectar.
- 1 tablespoon apple cider vinegar.
- 1 tablespoon extra-virgin olive oil.
- A pinch of black pepper.

Here are the directions for making this salad:

1. Toss the salad greens and onions together.
2. Whisk the pear nectar, vinegar, olive oil and black pepper together.
3. Add the dressing to the salad and toss until coated.
4. Sprinkle walnuts over the top of the salad.

5. Arrange the pear slices neatly on top of the salad.
6. Serve chilled.

Blueberry Pomegranate Smoothe

We've already discussed the potential anticancer benefits of blueberries. The same anthocyanins that fight cancer have been shown in a laboratory setting to dial down an enzyme that produces cholesterol. This experiment was run on hamsters, so it's unclear whether it has the same effect on humans (28).

Pomegranate juice has been shown to lower total cholesterol. A study of type II diabetic patients found concentrated pomegranate juice lowers total cholesterol and LDL cholesterol and the results led researchers to conclude consumption "could modify heart disease risk factors" and "its inclusion in their diets may be beneficial" (29).

Here are the ingredients you're going to need to make this smoothie:

- 1 cup frozen blueberries.
- 1 cup 100% pomegranate juice.
- ½ cup nonfat vanilla yogurt.
- 1 teaspoon lemon juice.
- 1 tablespoon apple cider vinegar.

Add all of the ingredients to a blender and blend until smooth. Consume immediately.

Cold and Flu Relief

Apple cider vinegar acts on colds and flus in a number of ways.

It relieves the symptoms by easing congestion and helping clear the sinuses. It kills the bacteria that cause sore throats and helps ease the pain. A hot compress can be made by mixing a cup of apple cider vinegar into 2 cups of hot water and soaking a towel or washcloth in it. Place the compress over your chest if you're congested or over your throat if it's sore for almost instant relief.

The internal workings of the body may tilt toward acidity when you're sick. Apple cider vinegar can help move the body back toward alkalinity. It can also be consumed to give your immune system a much needed boost that might help your body fight off the bug causing the illness. If you aren't already taking apple cider vinegar, the best time to take it is as soon as you first feel the illness coming on .

Cold-Buster Tea

Here's a recipe that combines a number of natural ingredients to help ease the symptoms of colds and the flu and to limit the amount of time you're down and out. Unlike over-the-counter cold and flu relief medications, this tea helps the body battle the cold or flu, instead of simply masking the symptoms.

Garlic packs a potent punch when it comes to cold and flu relief because it's antibacterial, antifungal and antiviral. It's able to kill drug-resistant bacteria and could be just what your body needs to fight off a stubborn flu or cold that won't go away.

Raw honey is soothing. It soothes the throat on the way down and helps soothe frazzled nerves. Honey contains antibacterial compounds that are able to help the body fight off some illnesses.

The capsaicin in cayenne pepper thins out mucus in the nasal passages and has anti-inflammatory properties. It also helps boost immunity, so you might be less likely to get sick after consuming it and it should help the body fight off illnesses faster than it normally would.

Gather the following ingredients:

- 1 cup filtered water.
- 2 tablespoons apple cider vinegar.
- 1 garlic clove, minced.
- 2 tablespoons raw honey.
- ½ teaspoon cayenne pepper.

Warm the water up and stir all of the ingredients into it. Don't get the water too hot or you'll kill some of the health benefits of the apple cider vinegar. Drink this concoction once a day until you start feeling better.

Hot Cider

Here's a recipe my grandmother used to make. She called it "hot cider." I've also seen it called fire cider. She claimed it helps you sweat out a cold or flu. I don't know how true this is, but it can make you sweat a bit. If you can handle the heat as the cider goes down, it may provide some relief. I don't recommend it if you've been vomiting, as I'd imagine it wouldn't feel very good coming back up. It also isn't a good choice for those who are prone to heartburn.

Here are the ingredients for hot cider:

- 1 cup water.
- 3 cups apple cider.
- ½ cup apple cider vinegar.
- ½ cup raw honey.
- 5 tablespoons grated horseradish.
- 4 tablespoons minced onions.
- 2 garlic cloves, minced.
- 2 teaspoons cinnamon.

Follow these directions to make hot cider:

1. Combine the water and apple cider vinegar and gently warm it up.
2. Place the rest of the ingredients (except for the honey) in a sealable jar and pour the warm vinegar-honey concoction over the top.
3. Seal the jar and let it sit for at least a couple hours.
4. Stir in the honey, to taste.

5. Shake the container vigorously before consuming.
6. Store in an airtight container in the fridge.

When you first start feeling sick, take 2 tablespoons once every 6 to 8 hours until you feel better. Be forewarned—this stuff isn't for the faint of heart.

Detox

We live in a poisonous world. There are toxins everywhere. We eat, drink and breathe toxic chemicals and pollutants on a daily basis. Many of these toxins never leave the body. They continue to build up until one day the body has had enough and starts to give out under the stress of carrying such a toxic load.

Detoxification can help your body rid itself of at least some of those toxins.

People often turn to apple cider vinegar as a detoxification agent because it is believed to help the internal organs get rid of toxins in the body. It's also capable of helping the body clear out fungal and bacterial infections and gives the immune system a much needed boost.

Vinegar Detox Drink

The following drink adds cayenne pepper, lemon juice, cinnamon and raw honey to apple cider vinegar to create a potent detox drink. The lemon juice helps detoxify the body and stimulates the liver, while the cayenne pepper kick-starts your metabolism and gets your circulatory system revved up. Cinnamon is thought to purify the body. The honey is there to aid with the taste of the concoction, but it provides health benefits as well. Raw honey is full of beneficial enzymes and antioxidants that can help the body achieve a healthy balance.

Here are the ingredients you're going to need to make the apple cider vinegar detox drink:

- 1 cup filtered water.
- 2 tablespoons apple cider vinegar.
- 2 tablespoons raw honey.
- The juice of 1 lemon.
- 1 teaspoon cinnamon.
- ½ teaspoon cayenne pepper.

This drink is best consumed warm. Gently heat the water and stir in all of the ingredients. Consume this drink a couple times a day before meals while you're trying to detox. Make sure you're eating healthy meals that consist of whole, raw foods. Your detoxification efforts will amount to nothing if you continue to eat unhealthy foods while attempting to detoxify your body.

Ginger Kale Detox Drink

Kale is one of the most strongly antioxidant vegetables there is. It's packed full of vitamins and minerals and is believed to naturally detoxify the liver. The fiber and sulfur in kale are also believed to help detox the body (30).

Ginger has both anti-inflammatory and antioxidant properties and is an herb many people turn to when it's time to detox. It's one of the most recommended ingredients in detox drinks in popular literature. Ginger is believed to work to detoxify the internal organs and to enhance the body's ability to cleanse itself.

Here are the ingredients you'll need to make the ginger kale detox drink:

- 1 cup water.
- 1 cup kale leaves, stemmed.
- 2 tablespoons shredded ginger.
- 1 tablespoon apple cider vinegar.
- Raw honey, to taste.

Place all of the ingredients in a blender and blend them together. Drink immediately.

Cleansing Lemon Drink

Lemon juice is one of the staples of the Master Cleanse, which is a popular detoxification program. While on the program, you basically drink nothing but lemon juice sweetened with maple syrup with a bit of cayenne pepper added for good measure. That, and salt water in the morning and herbal laxative tea at night to clean out your system. Advanced cleansers have been known to cleanse for 10 days or longer.

While experts sometimes question the health value of the Master Cleanse, there may be something to using lemon juice to detoxify the body.

Lemon juice helps alkalize the body, tilting the scale in favor of good health. This alone would be enough to make the body more efficient in clearing out toxins, but alkalinity isn't the only trick lemon juice has up its sleeve. It also contains enzymes that aid with digestion and is believed to purify the blood while acting as a scavenger of free radicals.

The cinnamon is added for flavor, but it also carries some health benefits. Cinnamon has been shown to regulate blood sugar and is used as a natural remedy for a number of illnesses and ailments. Cassia cinnamon is the best kind of cinnamon for this beverage, as it's the one that's been studied the most. Be aware that high doses of cinnamon may be toxic.

Here are the ingredients needed to make the cleansing lemon drink:

- ½ cup fresh lemon juice.
- 1 cup filtered water.
- 1 teaspoon cinnamon.
- 1 tablespoon apple cider vinegar.
- Raw honey or pure maple syrup, to taste.

Combine all of the ingredients in a cup and stir them together. Drink immediately.

Digestive Health

The human body is designed to function as a whole, not as individual parts, so illness or imbalances in one area can impact the entire body. As such, the health of your gut plays a huge role in determining your overall health. An unhealthy gut doesn't just cause digestive issues; it can cause health problems all over the body, as the body is unable to protect itself from illness and inflammation.

An unhealthy gut doesn't contain the probiotic bacteria and digestive enzymes it needs to properly break down and digest foods. This can result in indigestion and other stomach problems, as the food sits in the stomach for longer periods of time than it normally would. It can also result in malnutrition, even when ample amounts of food are eaten, because the body is unable to properly pull the nutrients out of the food.

While digestive issues and malnutrition are fairly easy symptoms to tie to gut health, there are a number of other health problems that can occur that aren't as easy to diagnose. The immune system has to go into overdrive when the gut is unhealthy. Since the body is wasting immune system resources on the gut, it isn't as likely to be able to battle other issues that pop up elsewhere. Immune system diseases, joint pain and even allergies can all come about as a result of poor gut health.

In order to restore an unhealthy gut, the probiotic bacteria and enzymes that are missing must be replaced. This is fairly easy to do, as all you have to do is start eating probiotic foods.

Here are just some of the many probiotic foods you can start eating to promote better gut health:

- **Acidophilus milk.**
- **Fermented vegetables.**
- **Kefir.**
- **Kimchi.**
- **Kombucha tea.**
- **Sauerkraut.**
- **Soft cheeses.**
- **Tempeh.**
- **Yogurt.**

In addition to probiotic foods, there are a number of supplements you can purchase that contain billions, or even trillions, of bacterial cultures in a single pill.

Apple cider vinegar also contains probiotic bacteria and enzymes that contribute to gut health.

Kombucha Tea

Here's a *kombucha tea* recipe that'll work wonders to boost your digestive health. Kombucha is packed full of probiotic bacteria that contribute to good gut health.

In order to ferment kombucha tea, you're going to need a *SCOBY*, which is an acronym for *Symbiotic Colony of Bacteria and Yeast*. A SCOBY is a spongy layer of cellulose material that is added to kombucha to ensure it ferments correctly. It adds the correct probiotic bacteria to the container and floats at the top, protecting the tea from outside organisms getting in.

Kombucha tea contains a small percentage of alcohol that comes about as a result of the fermentation process. It's usually less than 1%, but kombucha left to ferment for a longer period of time than recommended will contain more alcohol.

First, gather the following ingredients:

- 1 gallon water.
- 1 cup kombucha tea (can be bought from the store).
- 1 kombucha SCOBY (available online or from some health food stores).
- 1 cup sugar.
- 8 teabags full of black tea.

Follow these directions to brew kombucha:

1. Add the water to a pot and bring it to a boil. Turn off the heat and add the teabags.
2. Stir the sugar in.

3. Let the tea steep until the water in the pot has cooled. Remove the teabags and discard them.

4. Add the cup of kombucha tea to the pot and stir it in. This acidifies the tea and makes it less likely harmful microorganisms will be able to grow.

5. Pour the tea into a large glass container (or multiple smaller containers). You're going to need a SCOBY for each container you use.

6. Place a SCOBY in each of the jars. It will usually sink to the bottom, but may eventually rise to the top.

7. Place cheesecloth over the mouth of the container and secure it in place with a rubber band. This will allow oxygen to circulate into the container while keeping insects and at least some particulate matter out.

8. Place the jar in a dark area of the house and let it sit at room temperature for 7 days. As the tea ferments, a new SCOBY will start to form at the top. It may bubble and/or attach to the original SCOBY during fermentation. The longer kombucha ferments, the more acid it'll have and the stronger it'll taste.

9. After a week, taste the kombucha daily and bottle it in an airtight container when it has fermented to your liking. The SCOBY and a cup of this tea can be saved to make your next batch of kombucha. You can continually cycle kombucha in this manner, so you'll likely only have to buy a SCOBY once. If you want to wait

a while between batches, place the SCOBY in tea and store it in the fridge. Swap the tea out once a month.

10. In order to carbonate kombucha so it has a light effervescence, leave the bottled kombucha sitting at room temperature for an additional couple of days.

11. Once the kombucha is carbonated, transfer the bottles to the fridge.

Kombucha tea is good for digestion and gut health on its own. Add a teaspoon of apple cider vinegar to it right before you drink it for added digestive benefits.

Kimchi

Kimchi is a Korean dish made by fermenting cabbage. It's packed full of probiotic bacteria that contribute to a healthy gut. It's an acquired taste, and most people don't care for it the first time they try it, but it does grow on you after a while. It helps to remember that it's full of probiotics and is good for your gut.

There are a wide variety of kimchi recipes in existence. Purists will see this recipe and decry the fact that salted shrimp or squid wasn't included. They can be added if you'd like, but were left out of this recipe in an attempt to make it accessible to as many people as possible.

You're going to need a glass jar that can be sealed airtight to make kimchi. Special fermentation jars are available that will allow you to safely ferment vegetables in an anaerobic environment.

Gather the following ingredients:

- 1 head of Napa cabbage.
- ½ cup green onions.
- 5 garlic cloves.
- 2 teaspoons unrefined sea salt.
- Filtered water.
- 3 tablespoons Korean red pepper powder.
- 1 tablespoon ginger root, minced.

Follow these directions to make kimchi:

1. Wash the cabbage and the green onions.
2. Remove the core of the cabbage and chop the remaining cabbage into large chunks.

3. Chop the green onions.
4. Peel and mince the garlic cloves.
5. Place all of the vegetables into a bowl.
6. Add the red pepper powder and the sea salt to the bowl and stir them in.
7. Cover the bowl and let it sit for an hour. The salt will pull natural moisture out of the cabbage. Bruise the cabbage by gently squeezing it to release even more water.
8. Place the contents of the bowl into the fermenting container. Add water to the container until it's covering the top of the vegetables. Remove any air pockets that exist in the vegetables.
9. Place a weight made from a non-reactive material into the container and press it down. The weight should be big enough to almost fill the container and keep the cabbage below the surface of the brine. Press the weight down until it's below the surface of the brine. Add more water at this time, if necessary. Leave an inch of airspace at the top of the container.
10. Place the lid on the container and seal it so it's airtight. If you're using a specialty container, follow the manufacturer's instructions for sealing the container.
11. Place the container in a dark area of the house and let it sit at room temperature for a week. After a week, check the container to see if it has fermented to your preference. If it has, move the container to the fridge to slow fermentation to a

crawl. If you want to let it ferment for a longer period of time, that's fine, too. Check it daily and move it to the fridge once it's ready.

Apple cider vinegar can be added to this recipe right before you consume it. It already tastes strong, so you're unlikely to even notice the vinegar is in there. I usually add a tablespoon of vinegar per serving.

Saurkraut

If kimchi is a little too much to handle, sauerkraut is another fermented cabbage dish that has a completely different flavor. It's lactofermented, so it'll contain the same probiotic bacteria kimchi has in it.

You're going to need a fermenting container to make sauerkraut.

Gather the following ingredients:

- 1 red cabbage.
- 1 green cabbage.
- 1 carrot.
- 3 tablespoons caraway seeds.
- 3 tablespoons unrefined sea salt.
- 1 tablespoon raw honey.

Follow these directions:

1. Wash the cabbage.
2. Remove the core of the cabbage and chop the remaining cabbage into large chunks. Discard the core.
3. Wash the carrot and peel it. Cut it into small slices.
4. Place the carrots and cabbage into a bowl.
5. Add the sea salt to the bowl and stir it in.
6. Cover the bowl and let it sit for an hour or two. The salt will pull the natural moisture out of the cabbage. Bruise the cabbage by gently squeezing it to release even more water.

7. Place the contents of the bowl into the fermenting container. Add water to the container until it's covering the top of the vegetables. Remove any air pockets that exist in the vegetables.

8. Place a weight made from a non-reactive material into the container and press it down. The weight should be big enough to almost fill the container and keep the cabbage below the surface of the brine. Press the weight down until it's below the surface of the brine. Add more water at this time, if necessary. Leave an inch of airspace at the top of the container.

9. Place the lid on the container and seal it so it's airtight. If you're using a specialty container, follow the manufacturer's instructions for sealing the container.

10. Place the container in a dark area of the house and let it sit at room temperature for a week. After a week, check the container to see if it has fermented to your preference. If it has, move the container to the fridge to slow fermentation to a crawl. If you want to let it ferment for a longer period of time, that's fine, too. Check it daily and move it to the fridge once it's ready.

Coleslaw

Not everyone is going to be willing to eat fermented foods. This coleslaw forgoes the fermentation, but includes apple cider vinegar, which should provide at least some gut relief. Cabbage is rich in dietary fiber, so it's good for the digestive system regardless of whether it's been fermented or not.

Here are the ingredients you'll need to gather:

- ¼ head of cabbage.
- 1 carrot.
- 2 tablespoons apple cider vinegar.
- 3 tablespoons yogurt.
- 3 tablespoons sour cream.
- 1 teaspoon lemon juice.
- ½ teaspoon Dijon mustard.
- ½ teaspoon pure maple syrup.
- Sea salt, to taste.
- Pepper, to taste.

Follow these directions to make coleslaw:

1. Wash the cabbage. Remove the core and shred the remaining cabbage or chop it into thin slices. The cabbage can be chopped in a blender or food processor, but be careful not to chop it too much. You don't want to blend it until smooth. If you want to make coleslaw that looks great, try using two different colors of cabbage. Light green and purple look amazing when mixed.
2. Wash the carrot and cut it into thin slices.

3. Add the vegetables to a bowl.

4. Combine the apple cider vinegar, mayonnaise, sour cream, lemon juice, Dijon mustard, maple syrup, salt and pepper in a bowl and whisk them together.

5. Pour the dressing over the coleslaw and toss until it's lightly coated with dressing.

Lemon Ginger Tea

Ginger is consistently seen near the top of lists of foods that are good for digestive health. It's supposed to be able to help with the following digestive issues:

- **Colic.**
- **Gas.**
- **Loss of appetite.**
- **Morning sickness.**
- **Motion sickness.**
- **Nausea.**
- **Upset stomach.**
- **Vomiting.**

A small amount of ginger goes a long way. Don't consume too much of it or you run the risk of indigestion and heartburn.

Fresh lemon juice is also able to help with a number of digestive issues. It can help with bloating, gas, constipation, diarrhea and heartburn and aids with digestion. Lemons are known to be antiseptic and can help the body clear out toxins.

Here are the ingredients you'll need to make lemon ginger tea:

- 2 cups water.
- 2 to 3 tablespoons shredded ginger.
- 1 tablespoon apple cider vinegar.
- 3 tablespoons fresh lemon juice.
- Raw honey, to taste.

Follow these directions to make the tea:

1. Add the water to a pot and bring it to a boil.
2. Place the shredded ginger into the boiling water and let it boil for 10 minutes.
3. Turn off the heat and stir in the honey. Let the tea cool.
4. Strain out the shredded ginger.
5. Add the apple cider vinegar and lemon juice and stir it in.
6. Serve over ice.

Energy

Energy drinks and coffee are vices people use to get through the day. Small amounts of caffeine aren't too bad, but the mega-doses you get in energy drinks and double shot cappuccinos are doing more harm than they are good. Too much caffeine can contribute to insomnia, muscle tremors and elevated blood pressure.

Most adults can handle the caffeine in a cup or two of coffee a day, but if you're getting a coffee beverage complete with sugar and whipped cream topping, it's the sugar you should be more concerned with. Some coffee beverage can contain well over 60 grams of sugar in a single 16-ounce drink. Energy drinks aren't any better. They often contain more than 60 grams of sugar per can as well. To put things in perspective, that's approximately 12 teaspoons of sugar hitting your system all at once.

Don't be fooled by the nutritional information on the label. That energy drink you're buying that says 24 grams of sugar on the label actually has 48 grams of sugar in the can. Manufacturers change the per-can serving size to 2 servings to fool people into thinking there's less sugar in their drinks.

You don't want to go sugar-free either, because the aspartame and artificial sweeteners used to replace the sugar can be even worse. Your body senses the sweet taste of the drink and waits for the sugar to flood in. It never does and your brain is left feeling unfulfilled. This can lead to overeating later in the day as your body pushes you to eat more.

If you have to have something with caffeine in it, a cup of black coffee with no sugar or cream is the way to go. You'll get your caffeine boost for the day and won't have to pound down a bunch of sugar and calories in the process.

Apple Cider Vinegar Energy Drink

Those looking for a boost without caffeine can turn to this apple cider energy drink. It combines apple cider with apple cider vinegar and adds a touch of cinnamon to create a drink that'll keep you going all day long. The best part is you can drink a second helping if you start to burn out mid-day almost guilt-free because it's a completely natural drink and a cup contains less than 200 calories.

Here are the ingredients:

- 1 cup organic apple cider.
- 1 tablespoon apple cider vinegar.
- 1 teaspoon cinnamon.
- 1 tablespoon raw honey.

Here are the directions:

1. Warm up the apple cider and stir the honey into it until it dissolves.
2. Add the cinnamon and stir it in.
3. Remove the cider from the heat and let it cool to lukewarm before adding the apple cider vinegar and stirring it in. Don't add it while the cider is too hot or you'll kill the probiotic bacteria in the vinegar.

Get Gout Out

Gout is an inflammatory joint disease caused when uric acid crystals form in the joints where bones meet. It occurs when there is too much *uric acid* in the blood and the body starts storing it away anywhere it can put it. Uric acid is usually processed by the kidneys and eliminated from the body, but some people have too much uric acid in their blood for the kidneys to process. When this occurs, the body has to figure out other ways to get rid of it before the blood becomes too acidic.

Uric acid is a created when the body processes an organic substance known as *purine* that's found in foods. Foods high in purine should be avoided by sufferer of gout.

The following foods are high in purines:

- **Meats.** Organ meats like kidneys, liver, tripe, brains and sweetbreads. Most meats contain moderate amounts of purines.
- **Foods made from meat products or byproducts will also contain purines.**
- Fish and seafood.
- **Whole grains are high in purines.**
- **Beer.**
- **Some vegetables.** Asparagus, cauliflower, peas and spinach all contain purines.
- **Lentils and beans.**

Purines aren't problematic for most healthy people and you shouldn't go on a low-purine diet unless it's recommended by a physician. It's when the body is unable to process the purines in food that they become problematic and gout can come about as a result.

Gout deposits can be extremely painful. Gout pain typically comes and goes, with episodes taking anywhere from a few days to a month or longer to clear up. In severe cases, the crystals can grow to a large enough size that they can be seen as lumps under the skin. Gout commonly occurs in the big toe and the joints in the hands, arms, legs and feet. The pain can be debilitating in severe cases.

The following things can be done to avoid uric acid build-up that can lead to gout:

- **Avoid foods containing purines like anchovies, organ meats and legumes.**
- **Don't overeat.**
- **Drink at least 8 glasses of water a day.**
- **Reduce stress.**
- **Stop drinking.**

Certain prescription medications, exposure to lead and some dietary supplements may put you more at risk of developing gout. If you're suffering gout and are in one of these risk groups, discuss your options with your doctor before making any changes. If your doctor attempts to prescribe water pills or diuretics to treat another condition, make sure you let him or her know you're predisposed to gout.

The alkalizing properties of apple cider vinegar helps your body fight off gout. It's believed to dissolve gout crystals and the boost it gives to your immune system may prevent gout from coming back. It can also be diluted with water to make a bath into which you can place painful joints. Add a cup or two of vinegar to a gallon of warm water and soak the area that hurts. Alternatively, make a hot compress using apple cider vinegar and water and place the compress over the affected joint.

Cherry Vinegar Juice

Cherries have been shown to reduce the risk of gout attacks. The following recipe combines the power of cherries with apple cider vinegar to break up gout crystals and keep them gone:

- 1 cup organic cherry juice.
- 2 tablespoons apple cider vinegar.

Mix the ingredients together and drink this mixture a couple times a day at the first sign of a gout attack. Try to avoid sweetened cherry juice when making this drink because sugar can contribute to the formation of gout crystals. If you have to sweeten the drink, use a teaspoon or two of raw honey.

Celery and Carrot Juice

Celery contains a bioflavonoid compound known as *apigenin*, which has antioxidant and anti-inflammatory properties. It's been used for many years in Chinese medicine to treat gout and a number of other types of arthritis (31). There haven't been many scientific studies done on celery and gout, but the ones that have been done thus far have shown positive results (32).

Carrot juice is a healing juice rich with nutrients. It has natural anti-inflammatory properties that can help reduce the pain and inflammation associated with gout.

The ingredient list for this juice is simple:

- 1 cup carrot juice.
- 1 cup celery juice.
- 1 tablespoon apple cider vinegar.

Combine all of the ingredients and drink immediately.

Weight Loss

I'm not going to lie to you and tell you apple cider vinegar is going to torch the excess fat off of your body as soon as you start drinking it. That isn't going to happen. What it can do is help boost your metabolism and possibly contribute to additional weight loss if you're leading a healthy lifestyle.

Since it helps control blood sugar, taking it with meals will likely suppress appetite by helping you feel full for a longer period of time after eating. A 2005 study found that people who eat bread along with apple cider vinegar feel fuller and more satiated than those who eat bread alone (33). Another study in Japan found regular daily consumption of vinegar reduced body mass index, visceral fat, waist circumference and body weight when compared to a placebo group (34).

Apple cider vinegar's ability to combat candida may also contribute to weight loss. People suffering candida overgrowth often undergo intense cravings for sugar and simple carbs. Limiting the levels of candida in the body will likely lead to reduced cravings for high-fat and high-sugar foods.

Vinegar isn't likely to perform any miracles when it comes to weight loss, but it can be used as part of a healthy diet plan and lifestyle. It won't melt the pounds away, but may gradually help those taking it lose more weight than they would have if they weren't taking it.

The handful of studies done on vinegar and weight loss thus far are promising, but a lot more research needs to be done before any solid conclusions can be drawn. Further research may reveal that vinegar works well for weight loss when combined with a healthy diet, regular exercise and a healthy lifestyle.

Chamomile, Honey & Vinegar Tea

Herbal teas act as mild appetite suppressants and help support people's weight loss efforts. They really come into their own when used to replace unhealthy beverages like soda that contain high fructose corn syrup and artificial sweeteners. Herbal teas also relieve stress, which is one of the leading causes of overeating.

The honey in this recipe helps mellow out the flavor of the vinegar. It also helps satiate the body's desire for sugar in a natural manner and may help prevent sugar cravings during the day. Don't overdo it on the honey. It's still sugar and too much can be harmful.

Here are the ingredients required to make this tea:

- 2 cups water.
- 2 chamomile tea bags.
- 2 teaspoons apple cider vinegar.
- Raw honey, to taste.

Follow these directions to make the tea:

1. Bring the water to a boil. Turn off the heat and place the two teabags in the water.
2. Let the tea steep for 15 to 20 minutes.
3. Stir in the honey and apple cider vinegar while the tea is lukewarm.
4. Drink immediately.

Grapefruit Juice

There's a diet called the grapefruit diet that's been around since the early 1930's and is still in use today by people looking to lose weight. It's purported to help dieters lose 10 pounds in just 12 days. While these claims are dubious at best, grapefruit juice can be consumed as part of a healthy diet and at least one study has shown it does contribute to weight loss.

In the aforementioned study, 91 obese patients were given placebo capsules, fresh grapefruit, grapefruit juice or grapefruit capsules three times a day before meals for a 12-week period of time. After the 12-weeks had passed, the three groups given grapefruit products lost the following amounts of weight:

- The fresh grapefruit group lost 1.6 kg.
- The grapefruit juice group lost 1.5 kg.
- The grapefruit capsule group lost 1.1 kg.

The placebo group had only lost 0.3 kg, so there's a significant difference in weight loss between the grapefruit groups and the placebo group (35).

Here are the ingredients you'll need to make fresh grapefruit juice with added vinegar:

- 5 large grapefruit.
- 2 tablespoons apple cider vinegar.
- Raw honey, to taste.

Here are the directions:

1. Juice the grapefruit.

2. Add the apple cider vinegar and raw honey and stir them in.
3. Serve over ice.

Simple Weight Loss Formula

Here's a quick and easy apple cider vinegar beverage that can be used to stave off hunger and help with weight loss. It contains a handful of ingredients known for their weight loss and detoxing abilities.

Here are the ingredients:

- 1 cup water.
- 1 tablespoon apple cider vinegar.
- 2 tablespoons raw honey.
- 1 tablespoon lemon juice.
- ½ teaspoon cayenne pepper.
- ½ teaspoon ground ginger.

Add all of the ingredients to a cup and stir them together. Drink immediately.

Additional Reading

I hope you enjoyed reading this book and found it helpful. The following book contains information on how vinegar and other natural cleaners can be used to clean your house:

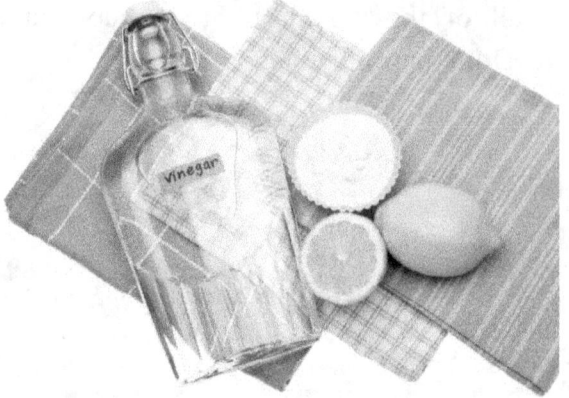

NATURAL green CLEANING

How to Clean Your Home Naturally

http://www.amazon.com/Natural-Green-Cleaning-Clean-Naturally-ebook/dp/B00H8IUPY8/

Here's a link to a book about probiotic foods that will help you add beneficial bacteria to your diet:

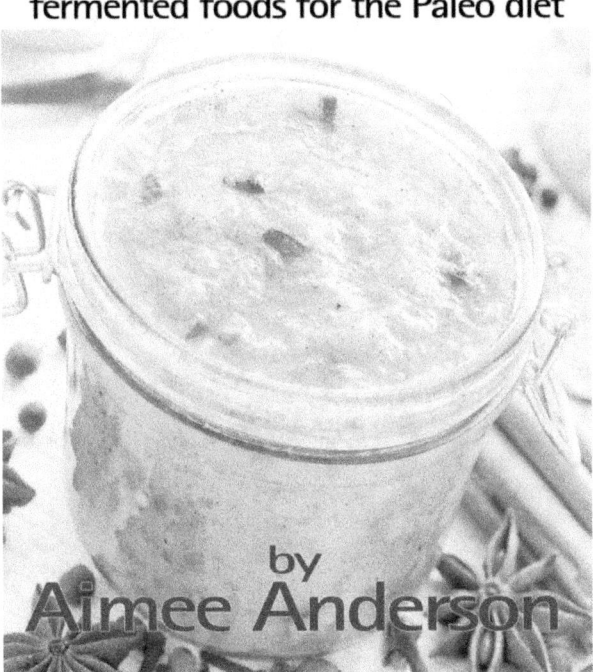

http://www.amazon.com/Paleo-Probiotics-Fermented-Foods-Living-ebook/dp/B00GYI4F08/

Here's a link to another Paleo recipe book. This one teaches you how to make Paleo bread that's free of gluten and is completely natural:

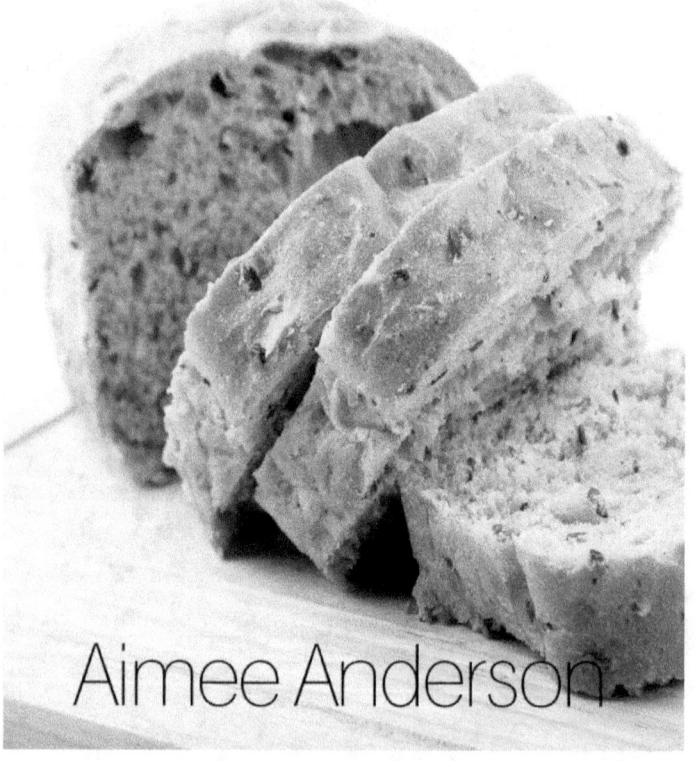

http://www.amazon.com/Paleo-Bread-Delicious-Gluten-Free-Recipes-ebook/dp/B00HFD2I1E

Works Cited

1. *Esophageal injury by apple cider vinegar tablets and subsequent evaluation of products.* **Hill LL, Woodruff LH, Foote JC, Barreto-Alcoba M.** 7, 2005, J Am Diet Assoc., Vol. 105, pp. 1141 - 1144.

2. *Nettle extract (Urtica dioica) affects key receptors and enzymes associated with allergic rhinitis.* **Roschek B Jr, Fink RC, McMichael M, Alberte RS.** 7, Jul 2009, Phytother Res, Vol. 23, pp. 920 - 926.

3. *Randomized, double-blind study of freeze-dried Urtica dioica in the treatment of allergic rhinitis.* **P, Mittman.** 1, s.l. : Planta Med, 1990, Vol. 56.

4. *Green tea: a promising natural product in oral health.* **Narotzki B, Reznick AZ, Aizenbud D, Levy Y.** 5, s.l. : Arch Oral Biology, 2012, Vol. 57.

5. 10 Natural Ways to Lower Blood Pressure . *Health.com.* [Online] 2014. [Cited: 1 1, 2014.] http://www.health.com/health/gallery/0,,20488689_2,00.html.

6. *Pomegranate juice consumption for 3 years by patients with carotid artery stenosis reduces common carotid intima-media thickness, blood pressure and LDL oxidation.* **Aviram M, Rosenblat M, Gaitini D, Nitecki S, Hoffman A, Dornfeld L, Volkova N, Presser D, Attias J, Liker H, Hayek T.** 3, s.l. : Clinical Nutrition, Jun 2004, Vol. 23, pp. 423 - 433.

7. *Potatoes reduce blood pressure in people with obesity and high blood pressure.* s.l. : American Chemical Society, Sep 8, 2011, Science Daily.

8. *Vinegar Improves Insulin Sensitivity to a High-Carbohydrate Meal in Subjects With Insulin Resistance or Type 2 Diabetes.* **Carol S. Johnson, Cindy M. Kim, Amanda J. Buller.** 1, s.l. : Diabetes Care, 2004, Vol. 27, pp. 281 - 282.

9. *Vinegar and Peanut Products as Complementary Foods to Reduce Postprandial Glycemia.* **Carol S. Johnson, Amanda J. Buller.** 12, Dec 2005, Journal of the American Dietetic Association, Vol. 105, pp. 1939 - 1942.

10. *Vinegar Ingestion at Bedtime Moderates Waking Glucose Concentrations in Adults With Well-Controlled Type 2 Diabetes.* **Carol S. Johnston, Andera M. White.** 11, November 2007, Diabetes Care, Vol. 30.

11. *Examination of the antiglycemic properties of vinegar in healthy adults.* **Carol S Johnston, I Steplewska, CA Long, LN Harris, RH Ryals.** 1, s.l. : Ann. Nutr. Metab., Vol. 56.

12. *Therapeutic effect of daily vinegar ingestion for individuals at risk for type 2 diabetes.* **Carol S Johnston, S Quagliano, S Loeb.** 1079.56, s.l. : FASEB Journal , Vol. 27.

13. How Does Fiber Affect Blood Glucose Levels? . *Joslin Diabetes Center.* [Online] 2014. [Cited: 1 12, 2014.] http://www.joslin.org/info/how_does_fiber_affect_blood_g lucose_levels.html.

14. *Activation of NF-E2–Related Factor-2 Reverses Biochemical Dysfunction of Endothelial Cells Induced by Hyperglycemia Linked to Vascular Disease.* **Mingzhan Xue, Qingwen Qian, Antonysunil Adaikalakoteswari, Naila Rabbani, Roya Babaei-Jadidi, Paul J. Thornalley.** 10, s.l. : Diabetes Journal, Oct 2008, Vol. 57, pp. 2809 - 2817.

15. *Commercially produced frozen broccoli lacks the ability to form sulforaphane.* **Edward B. Dosz, Elizabeth J. Hurley.** 2, s.l. : Journal of Functional Foods, Apr 2013, Vol. 5, pp. 987 - 990.

16. *Cooking method significantly effects glucosinolate content and sulforaphane production in broccoli florets.* **R. B. Jones, C. L. Frisina, S. Winkler, M. Imsic, R. B. Tomkins.** s.l. : Food Chemistry, Apr 18, 2010.

17. *Induction of apoptosis in human leukemia cells by naturally fermented sugar cane vinegar (kibizu) of Amami Ohshima Island.* **Mimura A, Suzuki Y, Toshima Y, Yazaki S, Ohtsuki T, Ui S, Hyodoh F.** 1 - 4, s.l. : Biofactors, 2004, Vol. 22.

18. Foods That Fight Cancer. *American Institute for Cancer Research.* [Online] Jun 28, 2011. [Cited: 12 24, 2014.] http://www.aicr.org/foods-that-fight-cancer/foodsthatfightcancer_green_tea.html.

19. Super Foods. *City of Hope.* [Online] 2013. [Cited: 1 13, 2014.] http://nationalevents.cityofhope.org/site/PageNavigator/wal k_super_foods.

20. Apples: A Healthy Temptation. *American Institute for Cancer Research.* [Online] 2013. [Cited: 1 26, 2014.] http://preventcancer.aicr.org/site/News2?page=NewsArticle &id=16477.

21. Cancer Studies. *Apples Prevent.* [Online] [Cited: 12 12, 2014.] http://www.applesprevent.com/cancerstudies.htm.

22. **Beller, Rachel.** Foods that Fight Breast Cancer. *The Dr. Oz Show.* [Online] 11 1, 2011. [Cited: 1 12, 2014.] http://www.doctoroz.com/videos/foods-fight-breast-cancer?page=2.

23. *Effect of Chia oil (Salvia Hispanica) rich in omega-3 fatty acids on the eicosanoid release, apoptosis and T-lymphocyte tumor infiltration in a murine mammary gland adenocarcinoma.* **Espada CE, Berra MA, Martinez MJ, Eynard AR, Pasqualini ME.** 1, Jul 2007, Prostaglandins Leukot Essent Fatty Acids, Vol. 77, pp. 21 - 28.

24. The Benefits of Fiber: For Your Heart, Weight, and Energy. *WedMD.* [Online] Nov 2, 2010. [Cited: 12 10, 2014.] http://www.webmd.com/diet/fiber-health-benefits-11/fiber-cancer?page=2.

25. *Nutritional attributes of traditional flaxseed in healthy young adults.* **SC Cunnane, MJ Hamadeh, AC Liede, LU Thompson, TM Wolever, DJ Jenkins.** 1, s.l. : Am J Clin Nutr, 1995, Vol. 61, pp. 62- 68.

26. **Staff, Mayo Clinic.** Cholesterol: Top 5 Foods to Lower Your Numbers. *Mayo Clinic.* [Online] Jul 27, 2012. [Cited: 1 23, 2014.] http://www.mayoclinic.org/diseases-

conditions/high-blood-cholesterol/in-depth/cholesterol/art-20045192.

27. **Weil, Andrew.** Q & A Library. *Weil Andrew Weil, M.D.* [Online] 8 27, 2009. [Cited: 1 27, 2014.] http://www.drweil.com/drw/u/QAA400608/Citrus-Pectin-Best-Bet-for-Cholesterol-Control.html.

28. *Blueberry anthocyanins at doses of 0.5 and 1 % lowered plasma cholesterol by increasing fecal excretion of acidic and neutral sterols in hamsters fed a cholesterol-enriched diet.* **Yintong Liang, Jingnan Chen, Yuanyuan Zuo, Ka Ying Ma, Yue Jiang, Yu Huang and Zhen-Yu Chen.** 3, s.l. : European Journal of Nutrition, 2012, Vol. 52.

29. *Cholesterol-lowering effect of concentrated pomegranate juice consumption in type II diabetic patients with hyperlipidemia.* **Esmaillzadeh A, Tahbaz F, Gaieni I, Alavi-Majd H, Azadbakht L.** 3, s.l. : int J Vitam Res, 2006, Vol. 76.

30. **Lewis, Alison.** Top 10 Health Benefits of Eating Kale. *Mind Body Green.* [Online] Apr 2, 2012. [Cited: 1 10, 2014.] http://www.mindbodygreen.com/0-4408/Top-10-Health-Benefits-of-Eating-Kale.html.

31. **Minton, Barbara L.** Celery Works Great for Inflammation, Gout, Cancer, and High Blood Pressure. *Natural News.* [Online] Sept 10, 2008. [Cited: 12 23, 2014.] http://www.naturalnews.com/024135_cancer_celery_inflammation.html.

32. Celery cures gout? *Best Gout Remedies.* [Online] [Cited: 1 23, 2014.] http://www.best-gout-remedies.com/celerycuresgout.html.

33. *Vinegar supplementation lowers glucose and insulin responses and increases satiety after a bread meal in healthy subjects.* **Ostman E, Granfeldt Y, Persson L, et al.** s.l. : European Journal of Clinical Nutrition, 2005, Vol. 59, pp. 983-988.

34. *Vinegar Intake Reduces Body Weight, Body Fat Mass, and Serum Triglyceride Levels in Obese Japanese Subjects.* **Tomoo Kondo, et al.** 8, s.l. : Biosci. Biotechnol. Biochem., 2009, Vol. 73, pp. 1837 - 1843.

35. *The effects of grapefruit on weight and insulin resistance: relationship to the metabolic syndrome.* **Fujioka K, Greenway F, Sheard J, Ying Y.** 1, s.l. : J Med Food, 2006, Vol. 9.

36. *Acetic Acid Upregulates the Expression of Genes for Fatty Acid Oxidation Enzymes in Liver To Suppress Body Fat Accumulation.* **Tomoo Kondo, Mikiya Kishi, Takashi Fushimi, Takayuki Kaga.** 13, s.l. : J. Agric. Food Chem., 2009, Vol. 57.

37. *Antihypertensive effects of acetic acid and vinegar on spontaneously hypertensive rats.* **Shino Kondo, Kenji Tayama, Yoshinori Tsukamoto, Katsumi Ikeda, Yukio Yamori.** 2002, Food & Nutrition Science, Vol. 65, pp. 2690 - 2694.

38. *Quercetin Reduces Blood Pressure in Hypertensive Subjects.* **Randi L. Edwards, Tiffany Lyon, Sheldon E. Litwin, Alexander Rabovsky, J. David Symons,**

Thunder Jalili. 11, November 2007, The Journal of Nutrition, Vol. 137, pp. 2405 - 2411.

39. *Dietary acetic acid reduces serum cholesterol and triacylglycerols in rats feda cholesterol-rich diet.* **Takashi Fushimi, Kazuhito Suruga, Yoshifumi Oshima, et al.** 5, s.l. : British Journal of Nutrition, 2006, Vol. 95.

40. *Protective effects of fermented rice vinegar sediment (Kurozu moromimatsu) in a diethylnitrosamine-induced hepatocellular carcinoma animal model.* **Toru Shizuma, Kazuo Ishiwata, Masanobu Nagano, Hidezo Mori, Naoto Fukuyama.** 1, July 2011, Clinical Biochemistry and Nutrition, Vol. 49, pp. 31 - 35.

41. **Yanjun.** Appealing health benefits of apple cider vinegar. *Natural News.* [Online] Aug 5, 2013. [Cited: 1 5, 2014.] http://www.naturalnews.com/041489_apple_cider_vinegar_health_benefits_natural_medicine.html.

42. **Wilder, Bee.** How to Overcome Candida Naturally. *Food Matters.* [Online] [Cited: 1 9, 2014.] http://foodmatters.tv/articles-1/how-to-overcome-candida-naturally.

43. **Young, Dr. Robert O.** *The pH Miracle.* 2003.

44. *Risk factors for oesophageal cancer in Linzhou, China: a case-control study.* **Xibib S, Meilan H, Moller H, Evans HS, Dixin D, Wenjie D, Jianbang L.** 2, Apr - Jun 2003, Asian Pac J Cancer Prev, Vol. 4, pp. 119 - 124.

45. 12 Natural Allergy Remedies that Provide Relief. *Reader's Digest.* [Online] [Cited: 1 25, 2014.]

http://www.rd.com/slideshows/12-natural-allergy-remedies-that-provide-relief/#slideshow=slide6.

www.ingramcontent.com/pod-product-compliance
Lightning Source LLC
Chambersburg PA
CBHW060405290526
45791CB00002B/614